D1859881

The Hindu-Yogi System of Practical Water Cure

Owing to the antiquity and rarity of this book, certain pages are regrettably absent, and readability is compromised due to the blurring of the original text. If you possess any insights regarding the availability of these missing sections, kindly inform us. Your assistance is crucial in ensuring the completion of this significant work for the benefit of future generations.

The Hindu-Yogi System of Practical Water Cure

As Practiced in India and Other Oriental Countries

BY YOGI RAMACHARAKA

GYAN

Published by

Gyan Publishing House
5, Ansari Road
Daryaganj, New Delhi-110002
Phone: 011-47034999, 9811692060
E-mail: books@gyanbooks.com

Distribution Network
gyanbooks.com
India, USA, Canada, UK, Australia

© Publisher

All rights reserved. No part of this work may be reproduced, stored, adapted, or transmitted in any form or by any means, electronic, mechanical, photocopying, micro-filming, recording or otherwise, or translated in any language, without the prior written permission of the copyright owner and the publisher.

ISBN: 978-93-6208-267-1 (PB)
First Published, 1909

2nd Impression 2024

Printed at: Gyan Press, Delhi.

The book is sold subject to the condition that it shall not, by way of trade or otherwise, be lent, resold, hired out, or otherwise circulated without the prior publisher's written consent.

THE HINDU-YOGI SYSTEM OF PRACTICAL WATER CURE
Author: YOGI RAMACHARAKA

The Hindu-Yogi System of Practical Water Cure

As Practiced in India and Other Oriental Countries

A Condensed System for Self Treatment

BY

YOGI RAMACHARAKA

London Agents:
L. N. FOWLER & COMPANY
7 Imperial Arcade, Ludgate Circus
London, E. C.

PUBLISHED BY
THE YOGI PUBLICATION SOCIETY
MASONIC TEMPLE, CHICAGO, ILL.

CONTENTS

CHAPTER I.

THE HINDU-YOGI WATER-CURE.

Among the Yogis of India, the system of Physical Well-Being known as "Hatha Yoga," in its many phases and forms, is followed, practiced and taught. Thousands of natives of India know no other form of physical culture, or methods of hygiene, and maintain health and physical vigor by an adherence to its precepts. In connection with Mental Healing, this system forms the great Natural Healing school of the Hindus. In our work on "Hatha Yoga," we have explained that system in general, and in many of its details.

There is one form or phase of "Hatha Yoga," however, which constitutes an important part of this great system of Natural Healing, which should be understood and practiced by those who would maintain a healthy condition of physical being, and which is worthy of being explained in detail in a supplementary volume—the Hindu-Yogi system of Practical Water-Cure. In response to many demands from those who were interested in our presentation of the general subject of "Hatha Yoga," we have incorporated in this supplementary book the details of the said system. We trust that we will bring to the attention of many persons of the Western world the benefits to be derived from this most meritorious system.

Water-Cure is not a new thing to the Western world. Many Western teachers have expounded its merits in a most forcible manner, and thousands of people have applied the method with excellent results. It must be confessed that both the Eastern and Western systems of Water-Cure have much in common so far as the actual methods are concerned, although the Hindus explain many of the therapeutic results by the theory of "Prana," which is unknown to the ordinary Westerner. An understanding of the principle of Prana in its phase of a therapeutic agent in connection with the Water-Cure, will throw much new light upon the entire system of the application of water to the cure of physical disorders.

"Prana," as our students know, is the great

universal principle of energy which premeates all things, and which has one of its manifestations in what is known as "Vital Force" in all living things. Prana is to be found in food, water, and air, in which three forms it may be used by living creatures and transmuted into Vital Energy, or Prana in its form of living force. In our work on "Hatha Yoga" we have shown how Prana may be obtained from food and thus transmuted and converted into vital energy and living force. In our work on "The Science of Breath" we have shown how the Prana in the air may be transmuted and converted into vital energy and living force. And in the present little work, we shall show you how Prana, which is contained in the water, may be transmuted and converted into other forms of energy, which will tend to invigorate and strengthen the human body, relieve physical disorders, and promote health and strength.

Of course, it is not necessary for one to believe in the existence of Prana in order to obtain benefits from the Water-Cure, for the virtue in the water is open and free to all, believer and unbeliever alike. But it is a known fact that when the mind recognizes the presence of Prana in the air; the food; and in the water; then there seems to be manifested a peculiar receptivity to its influence which is lacking to those who are not familiar with its presence. There is a good reason for this, but we shall not attempt to explain it here, for to do so would carry us into the realm of mental cause and effect, which is foreign to the purpose and scope of this little work. We shall, therefore, content ourselves with calling your attention to the presence of Prana, and the effects it produces when properly applied, and then leave the subject for the actual test and practical test of the student.

Prana permeates every drop of water, although in varying degrees. Fresh running water contains a much greater proportion of Prana than stagnant, still water. Likewise water that has been contained in cisterns, tanks, or vessels is found to have parted with much of its original store of Prana. And water that has been boiled has lost much of its Prana. This lost Prana may be restored by passing the water through the air, by pouring it from one vessel to another in order to "aereate" it. Distilled water usually loses much of its Prana, which may, however, be restored to it by pouring it from one vessel to another, through the air, as aforesaid. An understanding of this fact will explain the reason why the ordinary distilled water seems to lose a certain amount of its "life," which is noticed by those who drink distilled water as a measure of health preservation. Boiled water always seems "flat" unless it be poured through the air and reabsorbs Prana. Western science does not explain these well known facts, but the Hindus understand its cause to be the losing or gaining of Prana.

In using water for drinking, it is always well to pour it from one glass or vessel to another, backward and forward, several times. Those who will practice this plan will discover a new pleasure in drinking water, and will notice a decided improvement in the resulting effects. Water thus "Prana-ized" will be found to have a slightly invigorating and stimulating effect absent from ordinary water. Persons who wish to rid themselves of the desire for alcoholic stimulants will find it much easier to do so if they will pranaize their drinking water. The water in the pipes of the ordinary city water-supply is deficient in Prana—this may be overcome by pouring and repouring, as above stated. A little experimenting will convince the most skeptical of the virtues of this plan.

In the same manner, when one wishes to take a hot bath, or to drink hot water; or to apply hot-fomentations, etc.; it will be found advantageous to Pranaize the water in this way before using. In the case of a hot bath, dip up the water from the tub, with a saucepan or similar utensil, a number of times, until you have invigorated it with fresh Prana.

In this work we shall endeavor to use the ordinary Western terms and explanations, so far as is consistent with the fundamental ideas of the Hindu Water-Cure. We have no desire to surround this valuable, practical and simple system with strange verbiage and unusual terms. We shall quote Western authorities to support our position, so far as is possible. The Hindus entertain many ideas and theories which seem strange and fanciful to the Western mind, and we purposely omit all reference to the same. We wish to hold the attention of the student to the practical methods of the system, in connection with its fundamental idea, and shall run no risk of leading him up the by-paths of theory and speculation. This is particularly desirable in a work of this kind, which will fall into the hands of many who are unfamiliar with the Hindu theories and who have no taste for strange and unfamiliar ideas, but who want, and need, the practical, actual methods and instruction on the subject. Those who wish to understand the "why" of the Hindu ideas and teachings, are referred to our other works on the general subject.

To the Hindu-Yogi, water is Nature's great Remedy—its great Restorative Force. He believes in its liberal application, internally and externally. He regards it as the milk from the breasts of Mother Nature, which she would furnish to her offspring. The lower animals recognize this through their instinctive faculties, but "civilized" Man in his arrogance of reason has seen fit to depart from Nature's simple ways, and seeks in less simple things the virtues which reside alone in Nature's original fluids. In the following pages, we invite you to listen to the simple teachings of the Hindu Yogis on this subject. Do not let the simplicity of the system prevent you from appreciating its advantages. There is virtue in simplicity—danger in complexity. Nature's best things are always simple, and "common." To re-discover this fact, Man has traveled many a weary mile of thought and experiment. The advanced thinker always finds his road leading "Back to Nature."

CHAPTER II.

NATURE'S GREAT REMEDY.

It is no wonder that man in his natural state instinctively recognized in Water a Natural Friend and Helper. The instinct regarding water runs back much further than Man—back through the lower animals—back through the lower forms—back through the plant life—back through the elementary forms of life such as the amaeba, monera, and other tiny forms in the slime of the ocean bed—back to the very beginnings of organic life itself. Science tells us that organic life originated in water, and has always shown signs of its place of birth. About eight-tenths of our physical body is made up of water, and the very cells composing the body are virtually and actually marine organisms—tiny aquatic animals in fact—capable of existence only when surrounded by a saline solution of water. Is it any wonder then that the instinct for Water lies at the very foundations of our sub-conscious life, and manifests in our conscious wants.

And the important part played by water in our physiological mechanism is none the less remarkable. Physiology teaches us that over one and one-half pints of water passes from the body in the shape of perspiration every twenty-four hours; and that during the same time nearly three pints of water are passed off in the shape of urine—two quarts and over in all. The important juices of the body are composed of fluids, of which water is the basis. Not only is the blood, which is the very essence of physical life, composed largely of water, but also the bile, the gastric juices, the pancreatic fluid, and the several other juices of the digestive organs, as well as the saliva, are fluids of which water is the basis. Man can go without food for a number of days, but deprive him of water, and he perishes quickly. Water is one of the most urgently demanded of Nature's supplies, and next to air is the one upon which the continuance of life is based.

And yet how many people—or rather, how few of them—have given to this subject the consideration justly due it. And how few have made an intelligent use of Water a matter of habit in their daily lives. We give to the study of irrigation of the soil much care, time and thought, for we recognize that that is a subject upon which depends the welfare of our crops, and consequently our material welfare. But to the irrigation of the body, we give little or no thought, and are apt to dismiss the subject as of little importance. And, more than this, we take the greatest care to see that our domestic animals are kept supplied with sufficient water to drink, and in which they may bathe—we recognize the natural wants of these animals, and yet we do not think of bestowing one fraction of the same thought upon the wants and requirements of our own bodies, which should be of at least as great importance to us as those of the domestic animals.

It is true that in the state of nature, man was not so foolish. There he followed his natural instincts, and drank plenty of fresh water and washed himself in the stream, lake, or ocean—not because he had reasoned it out, but merely because he "felt like it," which was the manifestation of his instinctive knowledge. But as civilization advanced, and man began to live away from nature, he began to neglect these instinctive cravings of his nature—it was too much trouble to attend to them, and much easier to put them off. In the country, however, where water is near at hand, there is not so much cause for complaint. If one has good water on the farm, or good springs scattered around near the fields, he will take the little trouble necessary to procure it, and will drink about as much as he needs. But in the large cities, where the water runs stale and warm through the faucets, and is consequently not so palatable, man will gradually get out of the habit of drinking normal amounts, and will lose his natural instincts and acquire a perverted "second-nature" which enables him to go without water without feeling the distress which a natural water-drinker would feel under the same circumstances. But Nature does not forget—she remembers, and resents the fact that she is not being furnished the proper amount of fluids that she needs in order to carry on her wonderful work. She takes it out on the body, by allowing it to shrivel up, and exist in an abnormal, unhealthy condition. And these abnormal conditions are many.

One is filled with surprise when he looks around and sees how many persons go through the day with a consumption of fluids far below the natural requirements. They take merely a sip or two of water, during the day, and their consumption of fluids consists almost altogether of what they obtain in coffee or tea, at meal times, and perhaps a glass of soda, water, pop, beer, etc., during the day. They turn their backs upon Nature's Fount of Life. Is it any wonder that so many people are suffering with constipation and congested colons? Is it any wonder that their bowels are clogged up with the refuse matter of their systems, when they do not irrigate the canals with sufficient water to carry away the debris. No wonder their bowels are like dry sewers, caked with the foul matter which has been deposited in them as the waste products of the system. Women particularly are the principal offenders in this respect, although it is difficult to say just why.

These water-famished people are troubled not only with constipation, but their livers and kidneys do not work properly. Their blood supply is below the normal, and they exhibit a bloodless, anaemic appearance, and tend to "go into decline" early in life. Others, from the same cause go about with dry skin (showing seldom a trace of perspiration); pasty, sallow complexions, and a foul breath. Some of them resemble dried apples, and one instinctively wishes that they could be put into soak to make them plump out and look a little natural. And of course, all the other parts of the body, particularly the nerves, respond to these abnormal conditions, and give out warning signs. If you will check off the symptoms of the trouble arising from a deficient water supply, you will have a list of a majority of the more common diseases. The troubles arising from constipation, alone, will make quite a long list—and yet, constipation is due almost if not entirely to a lack of fluids, in one form or another, as we shall see as we proceed with this book.

Man's body is a great water-system, with pipes, large and small running in all directions, designed for the passage of fluids from one part of the body to another—fluids of which water is the base, remember. And there is only one way in which the supply of water naturally flows into the body—the alimentary canal, from which the water is absorbed and carried to all parts of the system, there to perform its wonderful work. Every organ of the body laves, bathes and lives in fluids, and without a proper supply they cannot function properly. Fluids dissolve the food and convert it into its various elements, that other fluids may carry it to the parts of the body where it nourishes and builds up the entire system, every cell demanding and receiving its share. Other fluids carry back the broken-down tissue, and waste-matter of the system, and expel it from the system by means of other fluids. It is all the work of fluids you see—no matter what chemicals these fluids may carry, the fluid medium is necessary, and the work of nature can not proceed without it.

The medicinal effects of water are well known. Water acts as a tonic, when taken internally and externally. In fevers the effect of water is quite well known, and it forms a part of the intelligent therapy of the day, no matter what the past history of medicine has been. Cold water scientifically administered as a drink, will reduce excessive heart action while warm water will increase the heart's action. Water increases the secretion of the kidneys, and helps that organ to excrete and dispose of the waste matter coming its way. It also acts in a similar way on the other organs of excretion.

Water is a splendid appetizer, administered properly, and at a right temperature. Hot water acts as a powerful stimulant, and also as an antiseptic. It also tends to rest the stomach, and as a sedative. In cases where a patient has lost a great deal of blood, by hemorrhage, physicians often inject a quantity of sterilized water, with a small amount of salt, into the circulation, which gives the heart something upon which to exercise itself, and which also takes up the weakened, and dying corpuscles clinging to the sides of the arteries and veins, giving them a fluid in which to live and move and work, and in other ways acting as a good substitute for the blood until the system is able to manufacture more.

As to external application, the uses of Water as a healing agent are most numerous. In this little book we shall have something to say about that side of the question, giving the reasons for each form of treatment, and the best methods with which to apply the treatment. We shall also tell you about "flushing the sewers" of the system, which alone are worthy of the careful thought and attention of every living person. We shall also have more to say regarding the use of water, in the way of drinking, so as to produce beneficial results. And, we shall have much to say regarding the use of water as a bathing material. All of these phases of the subject are interesting, and important, and we trust that each and every reader of this book will give to this subject the careful attention that it certainly deserves. Do not let the apparent simplicity of the thing cause you to discard it in favor of some more expensive, complicated and little-understood method or form of treatment. Remember, that he who sticks close to Mother Nature will receive the benefit of the methods which formulated by those universal laws which underlie all of the wonderful work of the cosmos, organic and inorganic. Nature is the Universal Mother—the Universal Physician—the Universal Nurse. You will do well to study her methods.

CHAPTER III.

WATER-DRINKING.

In the preceding chapter, we called your attention to the important part played by water in the physiological processes of the human system. We showed you that eighty per cent of the human body is composed of water, and that the work of the system depends largely upon water. We showed you that the healthy human being passes off in the shape of urine, perspiration etc., over two quarts of water every twenty-four hours. Now stop at this point and consider a moment. Over two quarts of water passed off every day—then where does it all come from? A portion comes from the liquid parts of the foods we eat, but the greater part must be placed in the system by means of water which we drink, else Nature is compelled to draw upon the fluids of the system for the deficiency, or else go on short allowance. If she draws on the fluids of the system, of which she has such a great store, the result is that sooner or later the body will become thin, and dried, and the person will lack sufficient blood and the other juices and fluids of the system—this is a logical necessity, for if the reserve is drawn upon, and is not replenished in like quantity a shortage must occur. But Nature generally compromises, and rather than deplete the body entirely of its reserve fluids, she compels the system to work on short allowance, and the result being that improper and abnormal functioning follows, and the patient suffers from a number of ailments, beginning with constipation, developing into dyspepsia, and ending in bloodlessness. And we see these people on every side of us, every day. If you doubt this, examine these rundown people, and in every case you will find that they take but a limited amount of fluids, while on the other hand, if you will examine the habits of the healthy people you will find that they partake of a liberal amount of fluids every day.

The best authorities agree that the normal amount of fluids that should be taken by the average person is about two quarts every twenty-four hours. Think of that you people who have been taking but a pint a day, or less! No wonder you are not healthy. How could you be, flying in the face of Nature in this manner. You must get back to Nature's normal conditions, if you would be healthy. You should begin by increasing your daily amount of fluids, adding a little each week, until you reach the normal amount. Do not gulp down large quantities at a time, but drink small quantities a number of times during the day.

You will find it an excellent habit to get into the way of drinking a cupful of cold water the first thing after arising in the morning, and another just before retiring at night. Then drink a number of times during the day. You will soon get back to the natural habit, from which you have strayed so long and so far. It may give you a little bother at first—the false habit may have become well established—but persevere, and you will soon regain normal conditions. Do not be afraid of drinking water at meal times—that old boog-a-boo has frightened off so many—the only thing to be avoided is that of "washing-down" the food. This "washing-down" habit is bad, for it prevents the thorough mastication of the food, which is necessary for a proper digestion, the saliva containing certain elements necessary for complete digestion. The water that you drink at meal times is quickly absorbed in the circulation and the work of digestion is not retarded thereby unless the water be icy cold in which case the stomach becomes chilled. So cultivate the TWO QUART PER DAY habit, and you will find that your constipated condition will vanish, and that your digestion will improve; and that you will begin to plump out again, and your cheeks will take on their rosy hue. You will have more blood in your system, and will feel better in every possible way. The water will be used in thousands of ways by Dame Nature, among others she will use considerable of it in the work of excreting and carrying off the foul waste products of the system, of which you will be informed as we proceed. This is the first great lesson of the Water Cure —TWO QUARTS OF WATER every day.

HOT WATER DRINKING. There is another form of water drinking which should be mentioned here—Hot Water Drinking. This method of cleansing the stomach has become qiute popular during the past few years, and formed an important part in the treatments of the original Water Cure practitioners. It acts along the lines of washing out the stomach; relaxing congested conditions there; loosening up the mucous accumulations, and dissolving them that they may be carried out of the system; and finally as a mild invigorator and stimulant.

Hot Water drinks should be taken soon after arising in the morning, or, if taken during the day, care should be taken not to eat for over one-half hour afterward. About one-half pint to one pint of water is the amount—taken as hot as it can be drunk with comfort, the usual directions being: "Make it as hot as a cup of hot tea." Hot water does not produce nausea—it is warm water that does this. There may be a little protest of the taste at first, owing to the "flatness" of the water, but this will soon be overcome, and many learn to relish the hot cupful. A pinch of salt may be added at first, if desired, in order to give a slight flavor. The water should be sipped steadily until the cup is emptied.

The Hot Water Drink has been used by many people with excellent results, and thousands of cases of indigestion, dyspepsia, weak stomach, etc., have been relieved thereby.

In addition to the advantages of Water Drinking recognized by the Western authorities, and which we have just stated to you, the Hindus hold that there is also a distinct and most decided therapeutic benefit obtained from the drinking of water charged with a full supply of Prana. In order to Pranaize their drinking water, the Hindus pass it through the air from one vessel to another, thus imparting to the fluid a new "life" which is quite noticeable, and which may be proven by anyone who will take the trouble to experiment with it. Water thoroughly Pranaized acts as a decided stimulant and invigorant, and imparts new vitality and energy when used in normal quantities. Who does not know the invigorating effect of a cupful of clear, vitalized spring water, or water from a mountain stream? There is a world of difference between such water and the lifeless water from the city water mains. And yet the latter may be Pranaized or vitalized by the exercise of a little trouble and work, in the direction of passing the water through the air in the manner just mentioned. If you learn what Pranaized water is, and what it will do for you, you will never be satisfied again with the de-Pranaized water used by the majority of people. In drinking Hot Water, be sure to pass it through the air as described, particularly if it has been allowed to come to a boil. In sipping water, allow it to remain in the mouth for a moment or so before swallowing. The nerves of the tongue and the mouth are those best adapted to absorb the Prana from the Water. Many Oriental people, recognizing this fact, often fill the mouth with water, when tired at work, and passing the tongue through it several times, then spit forth the water. They do not need the fluid as a drink, but merely wish to obtain its Prana. Try this sometimes, to prove it for yourself. But, do not neglect the drinking of a normal amount of fluids, for the majority of the Western people are deficient in this respect, whereas the Oriental always drinks his normal amount of fluids, having been accustomed to the same from early childhood.

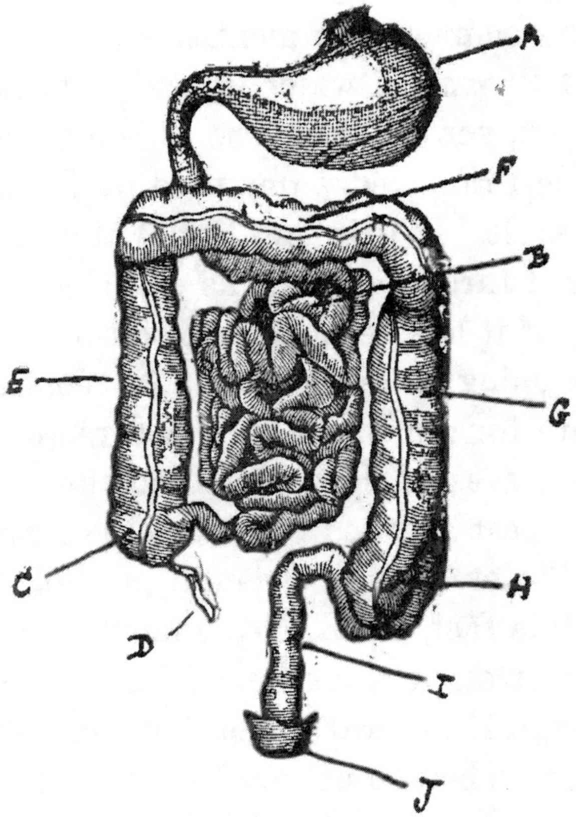

DIAGRAM OF STOMACH AND INTESTINES.

A. Stomach.
B. Small Intestines.
C. Caecum.
D. Vermiform Appendix.
E. Ascending Colon.
F. Transverse Colon.
G. Descending Colon.
H. Sigmoid Flexure.
I. Rectum.
J. Anus.

CHAPTER IV.

THE STOMACH AND INTESTINES.

We ask the reader to carefully study the accompanying Diagram of the Stomach and Intestines, for we shall have much to say regarding them in this little book. The student who will take the trouble to refer to the diagram will be able to understand the theories and practice referred to herein, much better than will one who merely glances at it and passes it by as uninteresting.

The majority of diseases may be traced back to troubles in the Stomach and Intestines, and the student who wishes to have a fundamental idea of the theory of cure of diseases, as well as the methods leading to such cures, should pay much attention to this part of the human system before he passes on to a consideration of other parts. It has been claimed that nine-tenths of the diseases and physicial disorders afflicting the human race have their rise and origin in this part of the system, and therefore it follows that if one acquaints himself with the normal functions of these organs, he will be able to construct for himself a working theory of treatment of conditions arising from an abnormal functioning of the same organs. Therefore we beg of you to read carefully the following brief description of the Stomach and Intestines.

Referring to the Diagram, and accompanying Key to same, and using the letters attached thereto, we begin at:

A. THE STOMACH. This organ is a pear-shaped muscular bag, holding over a quart. The food enters the stomach, after being chewed by the teeth; manipulated by the lips, tongue and cheeks; and moistened and softened by the saliva, which fluid also has a chemical action on the food, changing the cooked starch of the food into dextrine, then into glucose. The mass of masticated and insalivated food reaches the Stomach by means of a tube called the gullet or aesophagus which enters it at its upper opening. The Stomach then begins to digest the food, by means of a fluid which it secretes which is called the Gastric Juice. The Gastric Juice flows out in great quantities, and produces a chemical action on the food-mass, which changes its nature by dissolving certain portions of it; releasing the fat and breaking it up; and transforming some of the albuminous material, such as lean meat, the gluten of wheat and the whites of eggs, into albuminose, in which form it may be absorbed. While this chemical work of digestion is going on, the fluid portion of the food-mass as well as the fluids which have been drunk has been separated from the solids and then absorbed through the walls of the stomach and taken up by the circulation or blood supply, and carried out of the system by means of the kidneys, skin, etc. While the digestive work is going on, the stomach muscles are busily at work "churning" up the digested food. Soon a gray, semi-fluid mass is formed, called Chyme, composed of a mixture of some of the sugar and salts of the food; transformed starch or glucose; softened starch, broken fat etc.; and albuminose. (The above description refers to a Stomach acting properly. In cases of Indigestion, Dyspepsia, etc., the Stomach becomes like a great yeast-pot, filled with a sour, fermenting and putrefying mass.) This mass of chemically changed matter, called the Chyme, then passes on through the Pyloric Opening or "Gate," into the Small Intestine, which we shall now describe.

B. THE SMALL INTESTINES. This important part of the digestive system consists of a long intestine, or tube, nearly thirty feet in length, which is ingeniously wound around or coiled upon itself so that it occupies but a small space in comparison with its great length. Its entire length is lined with a soft velvety covering, arranged in a peculiar way that resembles plush, the appearance being caused by numerous small elevations known as the intestinal villi, which act as absorbents, secretents, etc. The Chyme which has just entered the Small Intestine from the Stomach passes along the thirty feet of velvety tubing, being subjected to the action of the bile, and pancreatic juices, which enter the intestine from the Liver and Pancreas, as well as the action of the intestinal fluids which are secreted in the Small Intestine itself. These fluids still further soften and dissolve the Chyme, and the chemical processes caused by their presence transforms the Chyme into three substances, viz: (1) Peptone, resulting from the digestion of albuminous matter; (2) Chyle, resulting from the emulsion of the fatty particles; and (3) Glucose, resulting from the transformation of the starch substances. These three substances are absorbed through the walls of the Small Intestines, and are carried into the circulation or blood-supply, and thence to all parts of the system. We have not referred to the part played by the Liver in this work, as our object is principally to follow the course of the food-mass through the Stomach and Intestines. After the valuable portions of the food-mass have been absorbed in the Small Intestine, the balance—the excrement, waste, refuse matter, etc., passes through a small opening, known as the Illeo-Coecal valve into the Large Intestine or Colon. This little valve is constructed quite ingeniously, in such a manner as to allow the excrement to pass freely into the Colon, but which prevents any of it from returning to the Small Intestine. Let us now follow this waste matter in the Great Sewer of the System—the Colon.

C. CAECUM. The Caecum is a large "blind end" of the Colon, just beyond the point where the excrement enters it from the Small Intestine. It is a rounded cavity.

D. VERMIFORM APPENDIX. The Vermiform Appendix to the Caecum is the little worm-like appendage which when inflamed gives rise to the trouble known as appendicitis. It is from one to five inches in length, and its uses are not known. Some claim that it furnishes a fluid needed in the work of lubrication, while others claim that it is the vestige of an organ which has outlived its usefulness in the course of evolution.

E, F, G, H, I. THE COLON. The Colon is the Large Intestine, or great canal, consisting of a large, membranous tube of about five feet in length rising as the Ascending Colon (E) on the right side of the abdomen; then passing over the Small Intestine, as the Transverse Colon (F); then descending down the left side as the Descending Colon (G); then forming that peculiar twist, curve, or knotty-shape known as the Sigmoid Flexure, (H), at the lower left-hand side of the abdomen; then passing into the smaller tube, known as the

Rectum, which is its terminal section, which ends in the Anus (J), or outer rear opening through which the excrement passes from the body. The Colon is the Great Sewer of the Body, through which the waste matter, refuse and excrement (known as "the faeces," or "faecal matter") is carried away toward the Anus, there to be expelled by a "movement" or "passage." When this great sewer is allowed to become clogged, the condition called Constipation ensues, and other evils follow in its train. The walls of the Colon contain tiny absorbent channels, which tend to reabsorb into the system the foul putrefying poisonous excrement, or waste matter, which Constipation prevents from passing along the normal channel, and which accumulates and chokes up the Colon, thus rendering the normally clean Colon the receptacle and retainer of a foul, putrefying mass. The absorbent capacity of the walls of the Colon has been proven by its capacity to absorb drugs that have been injected into it, the effects being manifested in a few minutes. Moreover, nourishment is often administered in this way, through the Colon, in cases where the patient is unable to retain food in the stomach. So you see that the Colon is capable of absorbing some very undesirable material back into the system, in cases in which it becomes clogged or obstructed. It is like the action of a sewer which "backs up" into your house drain-pipes, when it becomes clogged or stopped. This fact is not realized by the majority of people, who fail to realize the dangers of the situation.

It is with the Colon, that we are chiefly concerned in this consideration of the Source of Disease. In our next chapter, we shall consider it in detail.

CHAPTER V.

THE OBSTRUCTED SEWER.

We trust that you will pause at this point, and earnestly consider our advice that you read, carefully, deliberately and intelligently, every word in this particular chapter. We ask this as a favor to yourself, for what we have to say herein is a matter which is of the most vital importance to your physical well-being. What we have to say is not pleasant reading, for the subject itself is most unpleasant. But it is for that very reason that we urge you to study carefully this particular subject, in order that you may remove its unpleasantness once and for all. We are going to speak to you about a SEWER that you have within you, and which you have allowed to become most foul, through ignorance of natural laws. You have been carrying around with you a sewer which has been poisoning your entire body, and which has given birth to a host of ailments, diseases and symptoms which have arisen to plague and distress you.

You doubt this do you—then read on. That sour stomach, dyspepsia, indigestion, heartburn and other symptoms of indigestion arise largely if not entirely from this clogged sewer. That foul, fetid breath, muddy skin, pimply condition, "strong" sweaty exhalations, yellow eye-balls, dry skin, furred tongue, feverish feeling, nervousness and many other symptoms, arise largely from this foul, clogged putrescent sewer that you have been carrying around with you unknowingly. You doubt this—then there is all the more reason why you should study what we have to say on the subject. Read to the end of this chapter, and you will see for yourself—you will doubt no more.

The Colon, among the majority of animals and persons living a natural life, is free from obstructions, and is evacuated by frequent natural passages. With the majority of people living our so-called "civilized life" however, the Colon is seldom kept in good working order, and it is estimated that of such people nearly seven-tenths suffer from Constipation in some form or other, to a greater or lesser degree. Reports from hospitals where autopsies have been conducted show that in about five hundred cases in which examinations of the colon have been made after death of the patient, but about fifty were found to have Colons in a natural condition. The majority were found to be greatlyclogged with hardened excrement. The Hindu Yogis have known this for centuries, and Western physiologists now admit the fact.

Even among persons who claim to have a natural movement every day, there is often a condition of impacted Colon manifested. As Dr. Forrest, an American authority, has written: "There may be a discharge every day, even more than one, and yet the person may be badly constipated. Bear in mind that, accurately speaking, constipation means a loaded colon. Now, if from one end of this packed organ a small quantity is discharged daily, the colon still remains full by the addition at the other end, and thus constipation is present and continues even though there be a daily discharge. The discharge is from the lower end of the colon only." And, as another well-known American authority has said: "Daily movements of the bowels are no sign that the colon is not impacted; in fact, the worst cases of costiveness that we ever saw, were those in which daily movements of the bowels occurred."

Medical writers have, time and time again, expressed surprise at the amazing capacity of the Colon for holding excrement. There have been cases known in which enough matter was stored away to fill several Colons of normal proportions. The walls of the tube were greatly extended and swollen out, and packed almost tight with hardened faecal matter. Cases are on record in which people have gone for several weeks without movements. A case is related in which the treatment of Flushing the Colon brought to light cherry stones swallowed four months before. We think of importance to call your attention to the following cases of impacted Colon, in which the frightful condition of the Colon of many persons is stated plainly. It is not pretty reading, but everyone should be acquainted with the conditions possibly existing in themselves, in order that they may be impressed with the importance of taking steps to do away with the abnormal conditions, and thus bring about a return of natural functioning and action, which will bring Health in its train. We advise you not to "skip" these cases, but to read every one carefully.

Dr. H. T. Turner, of Walla Walla, Wash., U. S. A., reports the following interesting case: "In 1880 I lost a patient with inflammation of the bowels, and requested of the friends the privilege of holding a post-mortem examination, as I was satisfied that there was some foreign substance in or near the Ileo-caecal valve, or in that apparently useless appendage, the Appendicula Vermiformis. The autopsy developed a quantity of grape seed and pop-corn, filling the lower enlarged pouch of the colon and the opening into the Appendicula Vermiformis. This, from the mortified and blackened condition of the colon alone, indicated that my diagnosis was correct. I opened the colon throughout its entire length of five feet, and found it filled with faecal matter encrusted on its walls and into the folds of the colon, in many places dry and hard as slate, and so completely obstructing the passage of the bowels as to throw him into violent colic (as his friends stated) sometimes as often as twice a month, for years, and that powerful doses of physic was his only relief; that all the doctors had agreed that it was bilious colic. I observed that this crusted matter was evidently of long standing, the result of years of accumulation, and although the remote cause, not the immediate cause of his death. The sigmoid-flexure, or bend in the colon on the left side, was especially full, and distended to double its natural size, filling the gut uniformly, with a small hole the size of one's little finger through the center, through which the recent faecal matter passed. In the lower part of the sigmoid-flexure, just before descending to form the rectum, and in the left-hand upper corner of the colon as it turns toward the right, were pockets eaten out of the hardened faecal matter, in which were eggs of worms and quite a quantity of maggots, which had eaten into the sensitive mucous membrane, causing serious inflammation of the colon and its adjacent parts, and as recent investigation has established as a fact, were the cause of his hemorrhoids, or piles, which I learned were of a years' standing. The whole length of his colon was in a state of chronic inflammation; still this man considered himself well and healthy until the unfortunate eating of the grape-seed and pop-corn, and had no trouble in getting his life insured in one of the best companies in America."

Dr. Turner afterward conducted an extended series of investigations along the same lines, with the startling result that he felt justified in claiming that fully seven-tenths of adult mankind were afflicted in a similar way, in various degrees. He found that the colons of a great majority of the cases examined gave results corresponding very closely to those observed in the typical case noted above.

A Chicago physician, in an article in the Medical Examiner, gives the following result of his investigations along this line: "The muscular coats of the intestines are circular and longitudinal. In the large intestine the longitudinal fibres are proportionately longer than in the small intestine. Their greater length permits the formation of cells or cavities which become the seat of faecal accumulations only too often unnoticed by the physician. It is undoubtedly a fact that these cavities in the colon contain small faecal accumulations extending over weeks, months or even years. Their presence produces symptoms varying all the way from a little catarrhal irritation up to the most diverse, and in some cases serious, reflex disturbances. When the cavities only are filled, the main channel of the colon is undisturbed. Occasionally a cavity will become greatly enlarged and filled with faeces, reaching even the size of a faetal head, being mistaken for an ovarian tumor or a malignant growth of some abdominal organ. The most common part of the colon to become enlarged is the sigmoid flexure and the caecum. (See the Diagram in this book.) Accumulations can occur in any part of the colon. The ascending colon is much more often filled in life than the books would lead us to believe; indeed it may be said that chronic accumulations are oftener to be found in the ascending than in the descending colon, which is also contrary to the assertions of the authors. When the accumulations are large, the increased weight of the colon tends to displace it; then the transverse colon may descend even into the pelvis. The colon may be filled in an adult so as to present a circumference of fifteen inches. These accumulations vary in density; they may be so hard as to resist the knife, and thus be mistaken for gall stones. The mass may be so enormous as to press upon any organ located in the abdomen, interfering with its functions; thus we may have pressure on the liver that arrests the flow of bile; or, upon the urinary organs, crippling their functions. Reported cases of accumulations almost exceed human credulity. Enough has been gathered from the colon and the rectum to fill a common-sized pail. Of course such enormous amounts occur only exceptionally; it is not to these that attention is particularly drawn in this paper, because where they are so excessive any physician can detect them by means of an examination by touch. It is to the minor accumulations particularly that we wish to draw attention, the accumulations that we see in the majority of people. Such people contend that the bowels move daily, but the color of their complexion, the condition of their tongue, and above all the color of their faeces, are enough to assure us that they are victims of costiveness.

"Daily movements of the bowels are no sort of a sign that the colon is not impacted; in fact the worst cases of costiveness that we ever see are those in which the daily movements of the bowels occur. The diagnosis of the faecal accumulations is facilitated by inquiring as to the color of the daily discharges. A black or very dark green color almost always indicates that the faeces are ancient. Prompt discharge of food refuse is indicated by more or less yellow color. Absorption of the faeces from the colon leads to a great many different symptoms, amongst others anaemia (or bloodlessness) with its results, sallow or yellow complexion, with its chloasmic spots, furred tongue, foul breath and muddy coat of the eye. Such patients have digestive fermentations to torment them, resulting in flatulent distension which encroaches on the cavity of the chest, which in excessive cases may cause short and rapid breathing, irregular heart action, disturbed circulation in the brain, with vertigo and headache. An overdistended caecum, or sigmoid flexure, from pressure, may produce dropsy, numbness or cramps in the right or left lower extremity." Thus does Western physiology verify the old Hindu-Yogi teachings of "Hatha Yoga."

As the reader will have seen by this time, the conditions that make the application of the Internal Bath a necessity, arise from a violation of some of Nature's fundamental laws regarding normal evacuations, brought on by the unnaturad habits of life that have followed in the train of civilization. Man in his natural state lives according to Nature. He attends to the calls of Nature, just as do the animals, and consequently he is free from the effects arising from the unnatural retention of excrement in the colon. He does not need the Internal Bath, for the conditions which the latter relieves do not exist in his case. But now that the unnatural conditions are so prevalent, it is important that Science shall come forward with a method which will remove the obstructions which have been allowed to accumulate, and at the same time to point out ways in which a recurrence of the trouble shall be impossible.

Perhaps the worst feature about an impacted Colon is that it becomes the breeding place for innumerable germs of disease which are absorbed in the circulation and which are thus carried to all parts of the body poisoning and infecting the various organs and parts. Eminent investigators whose attention has been directed toward this important subject, have discovered that a majority of the abnormal and diseased conditions of the human system, which manifest as the various "diseases" (which are really symptoms of one fundamental cause), have their origin in these poisonous germs arising from the putrid excrement impacted in the Colon, as we have stated above. These germs have been generated in the foul breeding place, and have been absorbed into the circulation and have thence passed to all parts of the system carrying in themselves the seeds of disease, decay and death. Therefore it follows that instead of treating "symptoms" it would be wiser to strike right at the root of the trouble and remove the conditions which have brought about the various ailments.

How can one enjoy health if he has within

his system a foul, clogged up sewer, which sends its poisonous influences in all directions, affecting every organ and part of the body. What would be thought of a city which allowed such a condition in its main sewers—a foulness which sent its poisonous sewer-gas and germs into every house in the town? Would not the people arise in their might and insist upon a thorough cleansing process and a subsequent method of preventing a return of a like condition? Then why should not everyone pursue a similar policy in regard to the foul sewer which seven-tenths of them are carrying around with them. The cause is usually to be found in ignorance of the true condition of things, and it is the purpose and intent of books like the present one to throw light upon this dark subject, in order that people may make haste to remove the existing abnormal condition, and return once more to a normal, natural condition of life.

It is more than the mere heavy condition and ordinary symptoms of Constipation that we are now urging you to fight. Far more—it is the infected blood supply—the tainted fountain of life. It is the clogged up Small

Intestine and Stomach, which arises from the fullness of the Colon preventing the ordinary passage of the food along the natural channels, which in turn manifests in Indigestion, Dyspepsia, etc. The food being retained in the Stomach and Small Intestines far beyond its natural time, is apt to ferment and throw off acid substances, which aid in poisoning the system, generating gas, and causing heart-burn, sour stomach, etc. The liver, kidneys, and lungs become infected and their action impaired. Fevers ensue, and the system begins to break down under the unnatural condition. Nature uses the kidneys and skin to eliminate as much of the impurity as possible, but sooner or later the kidneys become overworked and broken down. The skin becomes muddy, foul and filled with eruptions. These things, and many others, arise from the clogged sewer—clean out the sewer and the various "symptoms" and "diseases" disappear. To sum up the whole matter, we would say that the Impacted Colon brings about a condition of POISONED BLOOD, and as the blood is the source of all physical building—the Spring of Life, as it were—you may readily see that if you will remove the poison from this Spring of Life, the vital fluid will run pure and free, carrying with it Health, Strength and Power, instead of Disease, Decay and Death. Is not this subject of sufficient importance to justify us in calling your attention to it so vigorously, and by means of the above startling and horrible statement of facts and actual cases?

And, now having pointed out the trouble, we hasten on to the method whereby it may be removed.

CHAPTER VI.

THE INTERNAL BATH.

The average person, once impressed with the truth of the statements and facts related in the preceding chapter of this book, would be likely to exclaim: "Dear me, I must get rid of this horrible condition at once—I must hasten to clean out that clogged sewer which has caused me so much trouble." Then, unless he be acquainted with sane methods, he will at once proceed to dose himself with purgatives, cathartics, laxatives, and what not—pills, powders, syrups, "waters," and so on, according to his lights, or want of light. Such is the natural tendency of people who have been brought up in a belief in medicines to "work their bowels"—victims of the Pill Habit. But this is not the right way—there are far better methods than these. Let us look at the matter a moment.

What is a Cathartic medicine? Some will tell you that "A Cathartic is a mild Purgative." But what is a Purgative? The definition is: "A medicine that purges." And what does "Purge" mean? The definition is "To cleanse the bowels by frequent evacuations." Well, that sounds good—"to cleanse the bowels." But does a Purgative Medicine actually "purge" or "cleanse"—and if so, how? To many this question may seem ridiculous, but those who have investigated the matter recognize the question as eminently proper, and know that the answer will surprise the majority of people. Let us see.

In the first place, the majority of people seem to think that a Purgative Medicine acts in some mysterious manner, by a power peculiar to and belonging to it, thus moving the obstructions from the bowels by its own force, virtue, and power. This is not correct, for the Purgative Medicine has no power of that sort within itself—it can move nothing by mechanical action nor even by chemical power acting upon the faecal matter. What really happens is that the Purgative Medicine contains within itself elements which are repugnant to the Stomach and Intestines, and which act upon them as irritant and objectionable chemicals. Nature, hastening to the rescue, and being desirous of removing the objectional and irritating substance, generates certain fluids which loosen up and lubricate the passages, and then cause a contraction of the walls of the stomach and intestines which force the objectionable matter from the system. The effect of the Purgative is caused by Nature's instinctive efforts to throw from the system an objectionable and harmful substance, just as it throws off and eliminates other poisons, by various channels, sometimes through the kidneys, sometimes through the skin—whichever way is the quickest and easiest, Nature uses to get rid of objectionable substances. The pain and "gripes" of Purgatives, are akin to the cramps accompanying the presence of poisons within the stomach—in fact, the Purgative is a kind of milder poison. Of course, in carrying off the poisonous Purgative, Nature also carries away a quantity of faecal matter which has become softened and lubricated by the secreted fluids. This is the whole story. But the impacted Colon is not cleansed by the process as we shall see in a moment.

The use of Purgatives is deplorable, in many ways. As a well-known English physician has said: "There is no habit so pernicious to the gastric digestion as systematically taking purgative drugs, and there is none more common." Purgative medicines irritate the stomach and intestines, and bring about a refusal of the parts to perform their normal functions in a natural manner. The Purgative Habit is acquired, and after a time the bowels practically refuse to act without the unnatural stimulus of the pill, syrup or aperient water. Besides this the action of the Purgative tends to cause Nature to secrete and excrete a considerable quantity of fluids in order to expel the objectionable drug, which in itself is a drain upon the system, as may be proven from the fact that extreme weakness often accompanies a violent purging. There could be no weakness arising from a getting rid of faecal excrement—the weakness comes from the unnatural drain upon the vital fluids of the system.

Besides the objections above urged against the use of Purgative Medicines, there remains another, and this equally important when the main object—that of getting rid of the accumulated debris is considered. As we have said in the previous chapter, there may be an apparently normal passage of the bowels without an actual clearing away of the impacted faecal matter. A person may have a movement every day, and yet be quite constipated. And a person may have just recovered from a severe "physicking" and still remain very constipated. For remember, once and for all, that Constipation means a choked and impacted Colon, and not merely scanty and difficult passages. Of course Nature makes a desperate effort to get rid of the waste matter, and in her striving she manages to keep open a small channel through the mass of impacted faecal matter in the Colon, through which the daily discharge passes. And when a dose of Purgative Medicine is taken the stream passes through this channel, washing away but little of the hardened matter. Clearly there remains something else to be done to get rid of this mass of hardened matter impacted in the Colon. There must be first a good, thorough sewer cleansing, before the after work of keeping the sewer free and clean is possible. And it is to this point that we have led you in our statements and explanation of the matter.

If you had a pipe, channel, or enclosed gutter badly encrusted with old accumulations of filth, what would you do? Wash it out with a hose, of course! The answer is simple. And when we ask you the question: What should you do to clean out that Great Sewer Pipe, filling nearly or quite half your abdominal cavity, possibly so distended as to be as thick through as your arm, choked, encrusted, and so packed full of hardened filth and foulness that its exhalations permeate your entire system, rendering your perspiration and breath so foul that it is plainly perceptible to others—how would you proceed to clean it out?" "Why, FLUSH IT OUT, of course, you stupid!" is your reply. Yes, that is the answer—FLUSH IT OUT! And that is just the process that is accomplished by the Internal Bath, of which we shall now proceed to tell you.

The principle of the "Internal Bath," or "Colon-Flushing," has received much attention from the Western writers and teachers upon the subject of Hygiene, and from the general public, during the last twenty years, and many had received wonderful benefits from an observance of its principles. Several persons, in different parts of America, have claimed to have made the discovery, but the chances are that they all worked out the problem independently of the others; and consequently all are entitled to the same degree of credit. As a matter of fact though, these "discoveries" were re-discoveries of an old principle well known to the ancient Hindus, and other Oriental peoples who practiced it centuries ago. Nay, more, it is believed that primitive Aryans received their first lessons on the subject from some of the long-billed birds of Oriental countries who are said to have practiced this method in order to relieve themselves of constipation consequent upon the eating of certain berries growing in those countries. One of the old writers insists that the method was learned from an observation of the habits of a long-billed bird dwelling on the banks of the Ganges, which was noticed to insert its bill in the water, and after filling the bill with a quantity of the fluid was seen to inject it into the anus for the purpose of bringing about an action of the bowels. Various species of the Snipe family are said to have similar customs. Pliny has written that this habit of the birds suggested the use of clysters to the ancient Egyptian doctors, and certain Chinese historians have claimed the same thing in their own country. So the practice seems to be universal, and having its origin away back in the early days of man's sojourn on this planet.

But there is a great difference between the ordinary Western methods of giving injections of water by means of the syringe, and the Hindu-Yogi methods. The ordinary Western methods consist of administering a small amount of warm water into the rectum, or lower end of the Colon, thus clearing away the debris from that region which had been clogging the lower end of the colon. This was an excellent thing, and far preferable to the practice of administering cathartics, etc., but the Hindu methods go much further, and accomplish far greater results. The "Internal Bath," which is often styled "Flushing the Colon," consists of the injection of from one to two quarts of hot water into the colon, thereby removing the mass of accumulated and dried faeces which have been poisoning the system, and which also has a tendency to give a mild flushing to the kidneys, as we shall see as we proceed.

Now all this seems so simple, that one who has not investigated the matter may be apt to consider that so simple and plain a process could not have been overlooked by Western physicians and hygienests for so many years, and that therefore "there must be something wrong about the matter." But, alas! like many other things it was too simple to have been thought of, particularly as the Western medical profession, up to twenty years ago, had not informed themselves regarding the dangers and frequency of the impacted colon. The few physicians and others who had acquainted themselves with the subject, were hooted down as quacks, and ridicule was meted out to them until a growing interest in the subject caused the profession to "sit up and take notice," and then investigation proved the soundness of the idea and method.

Many of the plain people of America who

followed the "Thompsonian System" of medicine, about sixty years or more ago, and who obtained splendid results by their system of "sweating and vomiting" the patient, thus getting rid of the poisonous matter in the system which had not been eliminated, and which caused the disease, also combined with their other methods that of the "large enema," or "injection" of hot water into the rectum and colon, by means of the ordinary syringe of that day. The amount injected was usually about a pint, but some of the more radical ventured to use a quart of water, which was quite unusual on the part of the medical profession and public generally, and which was regarded as a "heroic treatment" frowned upon by the regular physicians. About 1850, or perhaps a little earlier, one Dr. Joel Shew, in his little "Water Cure Manual," recommended the full injection. He said, among other things on the subject: "By a thorough washing out of the lower bowels, the peristaltic or downward action of the whole alimentary canal is promoted, and by the absorption or transudation of water, its contents are moistened or diluted and the whole of the abdominal circulation completely suffused by that blandest and most soothing of all fluids—pure water." And even before that time—say about 1825, Dr. Priessnitz, the eminent "Water Cure" advocate and practitioner, mentioned this among other subjects, as having produced the most satisfactory results.

But, these earlier practictioners and writers do not seem to have discovered the fundamental Hindu idea—the frequency and danger of the Impacted Colon. Their methods were directed toward the lower end of the Colon, particularly the Sigmoid Flexure, that peculiar curve or twist of the Colon just before it terminates in the Rectum. (See Diagram.) And so their methods, while excellent in so far as they went, did not reach the real source of the trouble, except incidentally. Perhaps the first Western man who really saw the value of the treatment and method was Dr. Wilford Hall, of New York City, a clergyman and scientist, the author of numerous religious, scientific, and philosophical works. Dr. Hall was broken down in health, and in his desperate endeavors to regain strength and health he experimented along many lines. Almost by accident his attention was directed toward the Colon, and he soon discovered the source of his troubles. He began treating himself, and the results amazed him—in a short time he was again hearty, well, strong and vigorous. Then he tried his treatment on some friends and acquaintances, with like results. Finally, feeling that such a discovery would benefit the general public, and having also the American business instinct, he published in 1880 his experience and his method in the shape of a small booklet, which he entitled "The Dr. A. Wilford Hall's Health System." He sold thousands of his "Systems" for prices ranging from $4.00 in the beginning, to $2.00 about ten years later. Through Dr. Hall's efforts thousand of families were made acquainted with the system of "Flushing the Colon," and others have since passed on the knowledge to others—but there are still millions of people who need this knowledge to-day and have never heard a hint of it! Another early teacher and practitioner of this method, was Dr. H. T. Turner, of Walla Walla, Wash., from whom we have quoted in the preceding chapter.

But, like many other valuable methods and systems, this one of "Flushing the Colon" was "overworked" by some of its zealous advocates, and turned into a fad. Some of the more radical advocates have gone so far as to claim that one should not bother about natural movements of the bowels, at all, but should rely entirely upon the flushing process, repeated once or twice a week, in order to keep clean the bowels. Now, at this point we wish to protest. We consider that a condition of that kind is as abnormal and unnatural as that brought on by the Pill Habit, and we advise strongly against any such fanaticism. There is nothing gained by getting away from Nature methods, and much to be lost. If men lived in the natural state, there would be no need for the Internal Bath at all. But, so long as they have allowed the unnatural condition of the Impacted Colon to be established, then they must use the next best method to remove the obstruction so as to allow Nature to assert her sway once more. And we know of nothing half so good as the Internal Bath, or Flushing the Colon, and that is why we so strongly recommend its use.

But after the normal condition is once re-established, then the person should lay aside the method (except for occasional use, as hereinafter stated) and should let Nature carry on her own work, aided and assisted by the use of the proper amount of fluids taken during the day in the shape of pure drinking water, etc., full explanation of which has been given in a previous chapter. So you see that we are not advising the constant use of the Inward Bath by means of Flushing the Colon—in fact we are urging the contrary. But before Nature can assert and re-establish her authority, the abused, choked, impacted, obstructed, encrusted Colon must be flushed clean and pure, and thus placed in a condition whereby Nature will be able to perform her natural functions.

HOW TO APPLY THE METHOD.

The method of taking the "Internal Bath," or "Flushing the Colon" is quite simple. To those who occasionally have administered to themselves, or others, the ordinary injection or "enema" practically no additional instruction is necessary. To those who never have administered an injection, a few words of instruction may be necessary.

Those who are familiar with the common form of injection, or enema, should remember, however, that there is a radical difference in the underlying theories of the two systems. In the old method of administering an injection, the idea was that there was an accumulation of faecal matter in the rectum, and in the folds and curves of the Sigmoid Flexure that lie just above it (see diagram). Consequently there was no necessity for injecting more than enough water to dislodge the obstructing mass—a pint being found sufficient for this purpose. The rectum and the Sigmoid Flexure may be cleansed by the injection of from one pint to one quart of hot water, in fact that is about their capacity, a larger amount rising above the curve of the Sigmoid Flexure. The old practitioners of the Water Cure doubted whether water could be injected above that point, except by a great pressure, and at any rate doubted the wisdom of attempting the same, their judgment being influenced by the belief that the clogging up was confined to the parts reached by their treatments. But the later investigators, recognizing the fact that the Colon could, and did, become clogged and encrusted along its entire length, and having found that much larger amounts of water could easily be injected into the Colon, until its entire length was flushed, began to increase the amount of water injected. Two quarts was the amount generally agreed upon as the proper average quantity, although some enthusiasts tried three quarts (after practice) and Dr. Hall went so far as to habitually use four quarts, or one gallon, in his regular treatments. But, personally, we do not approve of these large quantities. We think that two quarts will do the work as well as more, with less inconvenience and discomfort. In fact, we suggest that injection of but one quart at first, adding a little more each time, until the full amount of two quarts is reached—at which point let the quantity rest unchanged.

THE SYRINGE. Any ordinary hand syringe will answer the purpose; a cheap one may be procured from the druggist at the outlay of not over fifty cents, the better grades costing more. But better results may be obtained from the use of a Fountain Syringe, which is suspended high above so as to get the force of the flow of water.

THE PROCESS. In the ordinary enema the object is simply to cleanse the rectum, and about a pint of water is injected, and then voided almost immediately sweeping away the hardened excrement with it. But in Flushing the Colon the object is to inject the water gradually so that it will mount up past the Sigmoid Flexure, and on to the other parts of the Colon, there to be retained for a reasonable time that it may soften and dissolve the hardened faecal matter.

THE POSITION. Use your own inclination and preferences in the matter of position. Some take the injection in a kneeling posture, while others prefer to lie down—in this latter case we suggest that you lie on your right side, this being the position indicated by the position and location of the colon.

THE INJECTION. Insert the injection point of the syringe in the anus—a little oil, vaseline, or soap will render this easier. Then allow the water to flow in gradually and slowly. If you are a beginner, you will experience an instinctive desire to void the water at once, but a little exercise of the will power will cause this inclination to subside, particularly if you check the flow for the moment, not withdrawing the injection point however. Then after a moment resume the flow. If the inclination to pass the water becomes too strong, you may discharge the water and what it carries away with it, and then proceed with the injection. A little practice will soon enable you to overcome this difficulty. As we have said, one quart is sufficient for the first trial. After it has been injected, remain quiet, in a lying position if convenient, gently rubbing and kneading the abdomen with the hands, this process tending to loosen the impacted faecal matter. The evening, just before retiring is perhaps the better time for applying the method, although some prefer the morning.

THE WATER. The proper temperature of the water used for the injection may be regulated by the "feel" of the hand—let it be as hot as the hand can stand without discomfort—about the same temperature that you would use in washing with "hot-water."

FINAL. In passing out the water, do not be in too much of a hurry. Let it take its time. You will find that at first it will seem as if it were all out, but a little later you will find an inclination to pass more, which may be assisted by rubbing the abdomen from right to left. Sometimes say ten minutes after you have concluded the operation, there will be felt a final inclination, and the last of the water will pass from you, particularly if you walk about a little. The first few times you flush the colon you will be surprised, and perhaps disgusted, to perceive the character of the faecal matter that passes from you. In some cases great lumps of old excrement will be passed, much of it covered with a green, coppery mould or rust—in other cases lumps almost as black as coal will be noticed—all of which will show you the truth of the statements herein contained regarding the old, hardened impacted faecal matter which has been poisoning your system.

EFFECT ON KIDNEYS. Some time after the flushing, you will notice that you will pass more water than usual from the kidneys, the water having passed from the colon to the kidneys by means of absorption. Some practitioners advise that after the final passage of the water from the rectum, you inject a small quantity of hot water, and retain it, the result being that it will be taken up by absorption, and the kidneys thus given a beneficial flushing.

MISCELLANEOUS NOTES. Some who have practiced this treatment have found that in cases of extreme constipation and congested colon, the addition of a tablespoonful of glycerine to the hot water worked excellent results in the direction of softening the impacted faecal matter, lubricating the walls of the colon, etc.

Many persons ask whether the treatment is not weakening. To such we say that the extended experience of leading practitioners have shown that it has a contrary effect, a marked feeling of increased vitality being manifested by persons taking the treatment, after they have restored normal conditions. It does not weaken the intestines, but restores normal functioning to them, by reason of removing the obstructing materials.

The natural question is "How often should

this treatment be applied?" The answer is that at the start it would be well to apply it three nights in succession; then three times more "every other night;" then three times more," every third night;" then three times more "once a week." After this time a normal condition will have been restored, and by following our instructions in the preceding chapter regarding the drinking of a sufficient amount of fluids, one should be able to keep his colon in good condition. To those who do not take sufficient exercise, or who are confined to in-door life much of their time, or who, in other ways, are unable to live naturally and normally, we would suggest the benefit of a monthly treatment to prevent future returns of the old conditions. It would be well to set some particular time of the month, say the first or the middle of the month for such treatment, as one is more apt to remember such a set time when it "comes around."

Some practitioners of this form of treatment, recommend that after the treatment with hot water is completed, and the contents of the colon fully evacuated, it is advisable and helpful to inject a small quantity—say one pint—of water of the ordinary cold temperature, into the colon for the purpose of invigorating the colon and adjacent parts. The tonic and invigorating qualities of a cold douche, or treatment, after an application of hot water, is well known, many persons always taking a cold sponge after a hot bath—the practice of the cold douche or shower, after the hot bath, being a well-known feature of the Turkish Bath also. We mention this for the instruction of those who may favor or prefer it—it is not necessary however, and may be dispensed with without loss.

CHAPTER VII.

THE SKIN.

The majority of persons familiar only in a general way with their physiological structure, are apt to think of the Skin as merely an outside covering intended by nature as an armor surrounding the tender tissues underneath, and protecting them from outside irritating and injurious substances and objetcs. But the skin has several functions all of which are important, and which are as follows:

(1) The protection and covering of the inner parts of the body;

(2) The conveying of sensations to the brain, along the nervous system, by means of the senses of feeling, touch, etc;

(3) The regulation of the temperature of the body;

(4) The excretion of waste products and matter of the system;

(5) The absorption of substances presented to its surface;

(6) The function of an accessory organ of breathing.

This combined functioning renders the skin a valuable ally, and accessory to the bowels, kidneys, lungs, liver, etc., and consequently a very important part of the system. The leading authorities speak of the skin as being a protection from injurious and hurtful substances, both within and without.

The skin is composed of two distinct layers, viz., (a) the Dermis, (also known as the Cuta Veris), or True Skin; and (2) the Epidermis, or the Cuticle, or Scarf Skin. The Dermis, or True Skin, is the deeper layer or stratum of the skin, and is composed of a dense mass of net-like meshes, in which lie the muscular fibers, blood and lymphatic vessels, nerve sweat glands, etc., and the hair with its follicles. It rests upon the sub-cutaneous tissue of the body, in which is contained larger blood-vessels, lymphatics, nerves, muscle and fat. The Epidermis, or Cuticle, lies over the outer surface of the Dermis, and consists entirely of cells, being devoid of nerves, blood vessels, etc. The Epidermis is constantly discarding or "shedding" its outer cells in the form of dry flattened scales, new fresh and live cells taking the place of the discarded ones, the supply being kept up by the Dermis which forms these cells and then pushes them upward. These cells of the Epidermis grow harder, dryer and flatter as they rise to the surface. Not having nerves, the Epidermis does not feel pain, and having no blood-vessels it does not bleed when punctured. When you feel the prick of a pin, and the wound bleeds, the Epidermis has been pierced and the Dermis reached. A surprisingly large number of the scales of the "scarf-skin," or Epidermis, are discarded and cast off every day of one's life. Thousands of these tiny dried cells fall from the body during twenty-four hours. They are so small that we do not notice them except when they are gathered in quantities. We notice them when they have been gummed on the surface of the body by perspiration, the oils of the system, etc., and then removed when we wash, when they roll off as we apply the wet hand or cloth. Surgeons and nurses who are treating a fractured limb, will tell you that when they remove the plaster-cast which has enclosed the limb for a number of days, they will find over a wine-glass full of fine powder which has been cast off by the Epidermis—the waste cells of which we are speaking.

Considering the first named function of the Skin—that of a protecting covering of the sensitive tissues beneath, we are struck with the wonderful work of Nature in this respect. It is wonderfully soft, and yet equally wonderfully tough—it combines the qualities of silk and leather. It is remarkably flexible, and yet equally remarkably resistant. It repairs itself rapidly, and although constantly casting off matter it as rapidly replaces it. It is an armor wonderfully adapted to its purposes.

Considering the second named function—that of the conveying of sensations to the brain, by the sense of feeling, we find another wonderful adaption of means to end. A moments thought will show you that the great variety of sense reports that we receive through the sense of touch and feeling are received through the skin. Millions of sensory nerves terminate in the skin, and it is through these that we "feel" things. Through them we are made aware that things are hard or soft; rough or smooth; and the quality and character of resistence offered by them. There are tiny spots on our skin which register heat and cold. Some respond only to cold, and some only to heat. Physiology teaches us strange things about these "hot spots" and "cold spots," which however form no part of our present consideration, and we mention the subject but casually in passing.

Considering the third-named function of the skin—that of the regulating of the temperature of the body, we find that it is beautifully adapted to this work. Its vascular mesh is so extensive that it is capable of drawing to it and holding, in cases of necessity, nearly half of the supply of blood in the entire body, thus protecting the surface of the body from the effects of extreme cold. The "reaction," or flow of blood to the surface of the skin, which we notice after taking a cold-water plunge, is an evidence of this function. And, at the other extreme, we have the functioning known as perspiration, one of the purposes of which is to keep the body cool in hot weather, by means of evaporation. The average person excretes over one and one-half pints of perspiration during twenty-four hours, the amount being greater in warm weather than in cold. In unusual circumstances such as the case of men working in rolling-mills, tending furnaces on board ship, etc., the skin sometimes excretes as much as two or three pints an hour.

Considering the fourth-named function of the skin—that of the excretion of the waste products of the system, we find another instance of Nature's wonderful work. The waste products of the system are eliminated through the bowels, kidneys, breath and skin. There are myriads of sweat-glands in the skin, the number being estimated at about three millions or over, the combined length of which has been estimated at about five miles. The debris of the system is carried from all parts of the body in the blood which returns through the veins laden with impurities. A portion of this impurity is burned up in the lungs and exhaled by the breath; another portion is carried off by means of the kidneys; and a third portion is carried off through the skin, by means of perspiration. When the kidneys are weakened, the skin is called upon to do much of their work, in addition to its own. The water of which the perspiration is composed, is filtered out of the blood in the veins by the tiny sweat-glands, which then carry it to the surface of the skin where it evaporates and is carried away. The perspiration is not noticed to any great extent unless the weather is very warm, or unless we are exercising heartily, in which case it gathers in drops on the skin, and we perceive it. Even then, if the climate be a dry one, we do not notice it very much as the air takes it up so rapidly; but where it is humid and the air absorbs it but slowly, we notice it very much and find it depressing.

When analyzed by a chemist, the perspiration is found to be filled with foul excrement, debris of the system, and waste products, very similar indeed to that excreted as urine. This old matter is poisonous, and nature is making every effort to expel it from the system. Where the Colon has been allowed to become obstructed, the perspiration becomes very foul indeed, as it is called upon to eliminate much excrement that should have passed off through the bowels. One readily may see how very important it is to keep the skin in good, clean condition, that it may do this part of its work properly. Cases have been known where the skin of men have been covered with a coat of varnish—in one case a coating of gold-leaf being applied to gild a boy for a holiday spectacle—and in every case death ensued. Many contagious diseases are contracted because the channels of excrement are allowed to become clogged and obstructed, and the foul waste matter accumulates and breeds abnormal conditions—this refers particularly to the colon and the skin.

Considering the fifth-named function of the skin—that of the absorption of substances presented to its surface—we shall not say much at this point. In the chapters relating to the Wet Sheet Pack, and similar treatments, we shall go into the subject of Osmosis, in its two phases of Exomosis, and Endomosis, in order to explain the reason lying back of these forms of treatment. We pass by the subject here, in order to avoid useless repetition.

Considering the sixth-named function of the skin—that of being the accessory organ of breathing, we find that the pores of the skin act in the same general way as do the lungs, although to a minor degree. The pores absorb a small portion of oxygen, and give out a portion of carbonic acid gas. Some authorities have estimated that the skin performs at least one-fiftieth part of the respiratory function. It is thought probable that the races which go about naked, or partially so, use the skin in this way to a greater extent than do the races which cover the body with clothing, in which latter case Nature has adapted herself to the new conditions, and relieves the skin of a portion of this work, thus throwing a greater amount on the lungs. It has been noticed that when the naked races first begin to cover the skin with clothing, many of them sicken and die, this tendency however becoming less after a few generations.

In addition to the six functions, above named, the skin also performs a function for its own well-being and preservation, in the direction of secreting and using an oily fluid for the purpose of lubricating and preserving the skin and the hair. In a natural state, or when the person is cleanly about the person, this oil accomplishes its purpose and is rubbed off or evaporated from the body. But in unnatural living, and uncleanly habits, this oil has a tendency to accumulate and gum up the surface of the body, also taking to itself the remains of the waste matter excreted by the perspiration, and thus forming an unpleasant, unhealthy and abnormal obstruction and accumulation on the surface of the skin, and more particularly in certain protected parts. A word to the wise should be sufficient.

CHAPTER VIII.

SCIENTIFIC BATHING.

The use of the Bath as a means of promoting, preserving and restoring health, has been known to the Hindus from the earliest ages. In fact, it may be considered in the light of a primal instinct of the race. The primitive Argon did not bathe in order to remove dirt from his body—that is, he did not do so consciously—he merely obeyed the instinctive craving for laving in the stream or river, or swimming in the lake or sea, that arose from the depths of his sub-conscious self. With him cleanliness was merely an unimportant incident of the bath, the prime factor being his desire to experience that glow and throb of life that comes to all normal, natural and healthy persons when they plunge into the water. The exhilaration that he experienced was the cause of his persisting in the habit. Taught to indulge this instinct from early childhood, he naturally "took to it," as, in the familiar saying, "just as a duck takes to water."

The ancients, as the developed in knowledge, recognized the therapeutic value of the bath, as well as its natural hygienic virtues. They saw that not only was the bath calculated to preserve natural conditions of the physical body, but that also, when intelligently applied, it was a potent factor in the treatment of disease. And, so when the Water Cure idea began to develop among modern people, the practitioners naturally went back to the teachings of the ancients, and revived the therapeutic bath as an important adjunct of their system.

The reader who has studied what we have said in a previous chapter regarding the Skin, will not need much additional argument or explanation in order to understand just why the bath is a necessary factor in the health of every human being. When you remember the important part played by the skin in the matter of elimination of the waste products of the system, you will recognize the importance of the bath in the matter of removing the gummed up and accumulated debris which has gathered on the surface of the skin, and in its pores.

Bathing performs the same service for the skin, that flushing the colon does for the large intestine—in both cases the water washes away the debris and waste of the system, carrying off the foul excrementitious matter, and enabling the organs of the body to function properly. And both methods act in very much the same way, and produce the same general results. By keeping the skin properly cleansed, the kidneys are prevented from becoming overtaxed, and natural functioning all along the line is rendered possible, particularly if the colon is kept in a normal condition. Many skin diseases, and similar complaints could be obviated by an observance of both the flushing methods and intelligent bathing and cleansing the surface of the skin. Besides these important purposes, the bath acts as an invigorant and an exhilarant, and tends to keep the spirits bright, and the mind cheerful, clear and sound. We shall now proceed to a consideration of the various methods of bathing, advocated by the Water Cure practitioners.

THE ORDINARY CLEANSING BATH. Many persons will smile when they see this heading, for they are apt to think that there is very little to be taught regarding the ordinary bath. And, yet, very few really know how to get the best results from the ordinary cleansing bath. In the first place, the proper time to take the cleansing bath is either in the morning soon after rising, and before breakfast; or else in the evening, some time after eating, and just before retiring. Persons should avoid eating just before, or just after a bath. A bath should never be taken less than an hour after eating, nor should one eat a meal in less than a half-hour after the bath. The temperature of the cleansing bath should be regulated to suit the feelings and pleasure of the person bathing. Nor should people take a bath when they are greatly fatigued, or when the vitality is low. A medium temperature is preferable, neither so cold as to chill one, nor so hot as to produce the feeling of great heat. Both cold baths and very hot baths have their purposes and uses—we are speaking of the ordinary cleansing bath now.

Having your bath at the proper temperature, either in a bath-tub, or some substitute for the same, slip over your hands two mits made of Turkish toweling, without thumbs, and plenty wide enough to give the hands free movement. (The mits may be purchased ready made at the drug stores, or in the large city department stores—but they may be made by the housewife who understands sewing, from an ordinary Turkish towel, or bath-toweling.) Dip these mits (on the hands) in the water, and then rub a piece of soap well between the palms, so that the mits become thoroughly soaped. Then getting into the tub, give your body a thorough scrubbing off from head to foot. Then after the scrubbing, throw off the mits, and give the body a good rinsing down and rubbing with the bare hands. There is no substitute for the bare hands in this process, for they seem to have some virtue of their own, and then they fit the curves of the body better than can any substitute. At the same time you may administer to your body a gentle form of massage, rolling and kneading the muscles and limbs, rubbing the abdomen. Then dry the body with a thick towel. It is not necessary to rub the body roughly in drying off, as so many do; a soft patting and pressing of the towel answers the purpose and does not irritate the skin as does the rough drying process. The waste matter and the dead scarf skin have already been removed by the scrubbing and rinsing, so there is no necessity for the rough work with the towel. A little mild exercise after the bath is beneficial. Those who have not easy access to the bath-tub, may pursue the above method by standing before an ordinary basin, having some proper material on the floor in order to protect it.

THE KNEIPP NON-DRYING METHOD. Father Sebastian Kneipp, an eminent Western Water Cure practitioner, who was a Bavarian priest, advocated a method of "non-drying" after a bath closely resembling a favorite Hindu method, which many of his followers have found beneficial. We herewith give it, for those who may fancy and favor it. Father Kneipp says on this subject: "After a cold application the body should never be wiped dry, with the exception of the head and hands and wrists. The wet body should be at once covered with dry underclothing as quickly as possible, so that the wet parts may be hermetically sealed. Then the outer clothing should be put on at once. This may seem to be a peculiar proceeding to the majority of people not accustomed to it, and such may fear that they will remain wet all day long, but if they will but make a trial of this method they will discover by experience the advantages and pleasant results of this form of practice. The result is at once perceived to be a most regular, equal, and speedy natural warmth to the system. It is like sprinkling a little water into a fire—the internal heat of the body soon converts the clinging water into a greater and more intense form of heat. One may prove this by a personal trial. But, we must add that we advise exercise to be taken, either a walk or else work, as soon as the person is dressed after the bath, and this must be continued until the person is perfectly dry and warm.

THE HOT BATH. The Hot Bath has its place, but should not be indulged in to excess. It may be taken with the water at a temperature of from 98 degrees to say ten degrees higher. It should be begun by a scrubbing off with the bath mits, as before mentioned, and then followed by a "soaking" in the water for say, fifteen minutes, or so. Then before drying, one should take a wash off or douche of water at a considerably lower temperature. The hot water opens the pores, and without the cooler application there is a danger of sudden draughts etc., in some cases, which the cool application obviates. If one takes a daily cleansing bath, or cold bath, he will not need many hot baths for ordinary purposes. Hot baths have a relaxing effect, reducing the pulse and respiration, relaxing the muscles, and softening the tougher portions of the cuticle, etc.

THE COLD BATH. The Cold Bath is a very invigorating application, and is used advantageously by persons in good health and of strong vitality, but is not advisable in the cases of very young children, weak women, or any one whose vitality has become impaired. The benefits of the Cold Bath have caused many to make it a kind of "fetish," and harm has undoubtedly been worked in some cases by the blind following of a custom intended for only persons of certain temperaments, conditions, etc. There is nothing more invigorating to a strong man or woman, of strong vital temperament and constitution, than a cold bath. Its exhilarating effects are far more beneficial than any other stimulant known to man. But to apply it indiscriminately to young children, growing boys and girls, invalids, persons of impaired vitality, and the aged, is very foolish or worse. The whole secret of the Cold Bath lies in the REACTION, and unless this is obtainable the bath is more harmful than helpful. Much of the trouble comes from a blind belief that the water must be very cold indeed—the nearer to iciness the better. This is all nonsense—the sane idea consists in adapting the temperature of the cold bath to the constitution of the individual at the time. Many who cannot take the icy-cold plunge, are able to take a moderately cold bath with great benefit, and pleasure. In fact, we may say that any bath below blood-heat (98 degrees) may be considered a Cold Bath, the degree of coolness corresponding to the vitality of the bather—the more vital, the colder the water, down to a limit which ordinary sanity will enforce.

Father Kneipp, before alluded to, was a great advocate of the Cold Bath, which he taught imparted a certain hardness and ruggedness to the system, which acted as a protection against disease. He said on this subject: "One of the purposes of the cold bath is that of hardening the weakened organisms, and thereby strengthening them to renewed activity. The want of hardening the system is the cause of the extreme sensibility to disease on the part of the present generations. The people in these times have become effeminate. They are weak and delicate; very nervous; having insufficient blood; weak stomachs and hearts; the number of strong, vital and vigorous people being very few and far between. They are affected by every change of the weather; the changes of seasons brings to them colds and chest troubles. Even entering, or leaving a warm room, from or to the outer cold, works havoc with them. It is easy to see what is the trouble, and what the remedy. In order to keep healthy one must be hardened against the outer influences of changing weather, temperature, etc. Most unhappy is he whose lungs, neck or head are injured by every wind, breeze, or storm, and who is obliged to consult the weather-vane the whole year around, to know whether to venture out or to remain indoors. The tree is indifferent to the storm and calm; the heat and the cold. In the wholesome open air it braves wind and weather, and is hardened thereto by its nature. Let a healthy man try our cold bathing, and he will become like the tree."

In taking the Cold Bath, or plunge, one should avoid having the water too cold, particularly if he is not accustomed to the cold bath. Better have it less cool at the start. If it is too cool for the system, the reaction is slow in coming. You may easily ascertain just what the proper temperature is for you, by a little experimenting, until you find a degree of coolness which does not shock the system too much, and which brings on a natural reaction speedily. The first incident of the Cold Bath is the "shock" which comes immediately the body is plunged beneath the water, or when the water is poured over the body as the case may be. This shock at first drives the blood inward, in retreat, and the surface of the body becomes quickly chilled all over. Then comes the reaction, when emerging from the water you rub the body vigorously, moving about vigorously and inducing the flow of the blood to the surface, which is called the Reaction. The Reaction comes with a rush, and you feel a glow all over the body, which is very exhilarating and which sometimes continues for hours.

Never take a Cold Bath when the body is chilled. The proper condition is that of a warm body. If you are chilled when you arise, you should warm up the body by exercise before taking the Cold Bath. Neither should one take a Cold Bath when exhausted or fatigued by hard work, or after mental exhaustion, for in such circumstances the system loses a part of its power to react. Therefore, early in the morning is the ideal time to take this form of bath.

There are two general ways of taking the Cold Bath. The first consists in plunging the body under the water at once, allowing it to rest there a moment or two, and then stepping from the tub and bringing on the Reaction, as above stated. Some vary this method, by kneeling in the tub, and rubbing the water over the upper portion of the body with the hands, wash-cloth, or sponge. The second general method consists in standing up in the dry tub, and pouring a pitcher or several of them, filled with cold water down over the body, over the back and chest—this is akin to the "shower bath." A substitute for both methods is found in what is known as the "Cold Splash Bath," which consists in putting but a little water in the tub, and then splashing and patting it all over the body with the bare hands, finishing off with the "cold pitcherful" as above mentioned.

In any case, the Cold Bath is a matter of short duration, and one should hurry through with it. About one minute should be sufficient for the actual application of the water—in the case of the cold plunge, less time is required, it being an almost "instantaneous process." Quoting Father Kneipp once more, we call your attention to that venerable gentleman's remarks on this subject. He says: "Many have anxiety and fear regarding the application of cold water, from which it is difficult to free them. They seem to have a 'fixed idea of the loss of warmth.' They argue that the cold must take away the heat and thus weaken them. But they forget the fact of the reaction in which the warmth returns. Intelligently applied, cold water does not deprive one of warmth, but on the contrary supports and fosters natural heat. Let me ask you only one question: If a weak man, rendered effeminate by a sedentary life, and afraid to venture out-of-doors in the winter time, is found to have been so hardened and strengthened by the cold water treatment that he feels a pleasure in taking walks even in the coldest weather, and without any feeling of cold, or fear of taking cold, or without any resulting cold, must not the natural warmth have been increased in him? Is this wonderful increase in resistance to cold all imagination and illusion, or deception?"

GENERAL INFORMATION. The Cleansing Bath may be taken daily or at frequent intervals. The Hot Bath should be taken not oftener than once a week; and in case one is traveling it will be found that the ordinary cleansing bath will remove the accumulated dirt, without the need of the Hot Bath. Hot Baths are too relaxing to be taken too often. The Cold Bath may be taken daily, or once or twice a week. Be sure to see that you do not have the water too cold—study the reaction as a guide to the proper temperature.

A HASTY HAND-BATH. For those who desire the cleansing effect and general exhilaration of the daily morning bath, but who are so situated that they cannot have access to the bath room easily, we recommend the following as a Hasty Hand-Bath, which is well worth trying under the circumstances. Take a basinful of water, reasonably cool, and dipping both hands in it rub the water over the entire body hastily, and then wipe dry. You will be surprised at the invigorating effect of even this mild application of cool water, and will experience a bracing up and invigorating effect that will delight you. It acts as a good tonic, and hardener, and has rendered many immune from their former tendency to "catch colds."

FLOATING THE INTERNAL ORGANS. An effect of the bath not generally known to people, is that of "floating the internal organs," which may be described in a few words. In the ordinary standing position, our internal organs hang straight down from their natural supports; and when we lie down they hang down in another direction. When we place the body under water, there is a changed condition, differing from either the standing, sitting, or lying position—one which it is difficult to describe. The peculiar buoyancy of the water, and its pressure upon the body from all sides, produces a peculiar condition, inasmuch as the internal organs, or rather some of them, notably the liver, lungs, intestines, spleen, etc., rest freely in the space allotted them, without pressure upon each other and are thus given a sort of rest and relaxation, which relieves undue pressure and also tends to readjust minor displacements, etc. This effect may be obtained by filling the bath-tub nearly full of water of a pleasant temperature—about the temperature of the body, and allowing oneself to float around easily in it for a quarter-hour or more—without exercise, scrubbing, etc.,—just a state of "loafing and inviting one's soul." It gives one a splendid rest, and "loafing spell."

FOOT BATHS. We cannot urge upon you too

strongly the importance of bathing the feet. There is a peculiar connection between the soles of the feet and the nervous system, which evidences itself by the sense of relief and nerve rest afforded by the application of water to the tired feet, particularly at night. More than this the excretory channels of the skin, in the feet, are large and apparently perform more work than those in other parts of the body, as is evidenced by the tendency of feet to excrete foul-smelling perspiration. For this reason the feet should be kept clean and "sweet." Attention to the feet will repay you for the time and trouble bestowed upon them.

PRIVATE PARTS. The "private parts" of the body, including the anus (or outer opening of the rectum) should be kept scrupulously clean, not only from reasons of ordinary refinement, but also because the health of these parts depend largely upon careful attention. It should not be necessary to say more on this subject here to intelligent people. The idea of "Purity" should be evidenced not only in the inner sense, but in the outer also.

CHAPTER IX.

PACK TREATMENTS.

In our chapters on the subject of Bathing, Drinking Water, etc., we have pointed out important methods of keeping the system in good, normal working order, which will tend to prevent abnormal or diseased conditions. In our chapters relating to the Colon, the Internal Bath, etc., we have pointed out a most important method of relieving the system of a mass of obstructing material which retarded Nature's normal work, and which tended to poison the system. In the present chapter we wish to call your attention to other methods of relieving the system of foul excrementitious matter which has clogged up the system, particularly the skin, as we have stated in a previous chapter. These methods act on the same general principles as the Bath, but are far more radical in their application, and produce a quicker result which is desirable in cases where diseased conditions are manifested.

THE WET-SHEET PACK. This is one of the oldest Hindu methods of Water Cure, and has stood the test of many years. Originally pooh-poohed by the regular Western physicians, it has now forced its way to the front even in regular practice, as all who are familiar with the methods employed at leading hospitals can testify. Its simplicity makes it a most desirable method of treatment, while its effectiveness is marvelous. The following directions will enable one to apply this form of treatment with the best results.

First, spread over the bed-mattress, or cot, several heavy "comfortables," or similar covering. Then over these, spread a pair of flannel blankets. Then over the blankets spread a sheet which has been soaked in cold water (ordinary temperature as it flows from the faucet, or if well water let it be of the temperature common in the warmer seasons, avoiding extreme coldness), and which has been wrung out lightly so as to avoid dripping. Then have the person (fully undressed and without any clothing), lie down on the wet sheet, on the flat of his back, and his arms at his sides. Then wrap the sheet carefully around and over him, until he is well enfolded in it. Then wrap the blankets around him, over the sheet, in the same way. Then wrap the comfortables around him, over the blankets, in the same way. He is now well wrapped up, like a mummy, in the three sets of wrappings. The head is of course let out, and should be raised up on a pillow, in a comfortable manner. Be sure that the feet are well wrapped and tucked in. If the feet do not get warm with the rest of the body, it may be well to apply a jug, bottle, or rubber-bag of hot water to them for a while. If the patient manifests a tendency to headache, apply to his forehead a towel which has been soaked in cold water, and then wrung out, which should be renewed as often as it grows warm. The usual time for the patient to remain in the pack is from thirty minutes, to forty-five. Thirty is perhaps enough at first, unless he finds himself perfectly comfortable and desires to remain longer. We do not advise longer than forty-five minutes, in any case, as by that time the benefit of the treatment will have been gained.

See that there is sufficient fresh air in the

room. If the patient falls asleep it will not interfere with the treatment. If the patient warms up very rapidly it may be well to limit the treatment, to say twenty or thirty minutes. There is a great difference in patients in this respect, some warming up rapidly, while others respond very slowly. The object is not to "sweat" the patient severely, as many have supposed, but to induce other physiological action, and a fair degree of "warmth" is all that is needed, although, of course, he will perspire more or less freely and thus throw off much excrementitious matter.

When the treatment is concluded, he should be washed down well with luke-warm water and soap, followed with cooler water, and a good rubbing down. He should be given cool water to drink before, and during the treatment, letting him sip the fluid, however, instead of drinking large mouthfulls.

If the patient is inclined to be weak before the treatment, you would do well to substitute a sheet which has been soaked in luke-warm water, instead of the cold-water sheet as stated above. Use discretion and common sense in this matter.

You will find that it requires quite a little practice and dexterity in wrapping the patient up properly, and it would be well to practice on someone, with dry sheets, etc., before you attempt the regular treatment. Unless the wrapping be done neatly, the patient will find it uncomfortable, whereas if the work be done properly he will feel comfortable and at ease, and will enjoy the treatment. A coarse sheet is better than a fine one, and you would do well to keep one or more on hand if you intend using this treatment in your family. The sheets should be well washed after each treatment, as they become filled with foul, sweaty matter.

This treatment has a peculiar effect on the system. It loosens the dead skin on the surface, causing it to "peel" off, and it also opens up the pores of the skin, allowing them to excrete freely and throw off the waste of the system. The water has a peculiar "drawing" effect, and brings to the surface the foul matter stored away far below the surface of the skin, very much as a salve which is applied to a boil "draws" to the surface the foul pus, etc. It is astonishing how much foul matter is thus drawn to the surface and expelled from the system in this treatment. If the patient is billious, or his liver has not been acting properly, or if his kidneys and skin have not been doing their work, you will find that the sheet will be stained a yellowish hue, and will give out an unpleasant odor. In some cases the odor is quite perceptible, and may be noticed by the persons in the room, and at times the sheet will be stained so yellow that it would seem that actual pus exuded from the person in his sweat. A trial or two will convince the most skeptical of the value of this treatment as a means of removing the foul waste matter accumulated in the system.

Dr. R. T. Trall, the eminent American pioneer of Natural Healing and the Western Water Cure, says on the above point: "If anyone doubts the purifying efficacy of the Wet Sheet Pack, he can have a 'demonstration strong' by the following experiment: Take any man in apparently fair health, who is not accustomed to daily bathing, who lives at a first-class hotel, takes a bottle of wine at dinner, a glass of brandy and water occasionally, and smokes from three to six cigars a day. Put him in a pack, and let him soak one or two hours. On taking him out, the intolerable stench will convince all persons present that his blood and secretions were exceedingly befouled, and that a process of depuration is going on rapidly." If a person is a heavy meat eater; a heavy drinker; or a steady smoker; the tell-tale sheet will reveal more than an average amount of excreted foulness, all of which tells its tale to the thinking person. It is a good thing for the person in ordinary "good health" to take a Wet Sheet Pack, say once a month, in order to get rid of the accumulated debris of the system. The condition of the sheet will show that he needed it.

THE HALF-PACK. This is a modification of the above mentioned treatment, and consists in an application of the sheet merely to the trunk of the body—that is, from the arm pits to the hips. It is used in cases where the patient is too weak and feeble to stand the effect of the full-pack.

THE SWEAT PACK. This is a modification of the first mentioned treatment, its principal difference lying in the fact that the patient drinks freely of hot water while he is packed up in the blankets. In this treatment, the patient is required to remain in the pack for at least an hour, in which time he will perspire freely. He should be washed off after the treatment as above mentioned. This treatment is rather severe, and many practitioners do not now use it, they having found that the ordinary Wet Sheet Pack, varied with an occasional Hot Bath, is preferable and produces the same or better results with less discomfort to the patient.

ENDOSMOSE AND EXOMOSE. In order that you may have a more intelligent and thorough understanding of the process by which the Pack Treatment effects its beneficent results, we desire to call your attention to the principles known as Endosmose and Exosmose. Both of these principles rest on the fundamental principle of "Osmose," which Webster defines as: "(a) The tendency in fluids to mix, or become equably diffused when in contact; (b) The action produced by this tendency, as where the fluids pass through an intervening membrane. "Endosmose" is defined by Webster as: "The transmission of fluid, or gas, from without inward, in the phenomena or process of osmose." The same authority defines "Exosmose" as: The passage of fluids outward, in osmose." So you see that both of the latter are but forms of the principle of Osmose, which is a manifestation of a law or principle of nature which causes liquids in contact, or separated by a membrane, to tend to mix or exchange positions. Physiology teaches us that when there are dissimilar fluids so placed that only a piece of animal membrane separates them, they begin to move to exchange positions, or rather to mix up so that in the end when the two sets of fluids become identical in substance and composition, the exchange ceases. To illustrate, if you place ink and water in a vessel, the two being separated by a piece of animal membrane, the two will exchange positions, and mix up until each become identical with the other; and both would be diluted ink.

Now, in the case of the Wet Sheet Pack, etc., the fluids in the body, and those without, tend to flow in and out and mix up, according to the above named principles. The blood in the small capillaries or tiny blood vessels having their termination just below the surface of the skin, is composed largely of water, and holds in solution the waste products of the system which Nature is endeavoring to expel by means of the skin, through the pores. Now, when the water on the Wet Sheet, (which is prevented from evaporating) is brought in contact with the membrane of the skin, with its many tiny pores, there is set up an interchange of the fluids within and the fluids without, according to the principles of Endosmose and Exosmose, as above stated. The impure fluids flow out to the sheet, and the pure water flows in, until an equilibrium is established between the without and the within. The warmth generated by the pack, also tends to loosen and open the pores and thus encourage the ordinary throwing off by the perspiration. A double result is thus gained, (1) the blood is supplied with pure fluid in place of foul, while the foul excrementitious fluids and matter are deposited on the sheet and soaked up by it, thus getting it out of the system with no possibility of return. In view of the above explanation, you will see readily why the Wet Sheet Pack becomes such a valuable therapeutic method, and why it is superior to ordinary baths or sweats—it accomplished the results of both at the same time, and in a more thorough manner.

Practitioners have noticed, that in the cases of people who take the Wet Sheet Pack treatment, regularly, say once a month, the skin gradually becomes soft, velvety, and beautiful; its texture becomes more firm and sound, and the pores seem to function more vigorous and normally. The wearing of the clothing which civilization demands, tends to cause the skin to lose its vigor and functioning power. In such cases, treatments such as the above, and intelligent bathing methods, tend to restore normal and natural conditions and functioning powers. We think that you will find that this form of treatment will confer many minor benefits, in addition to the major ones herein mentioned. Try it, and see for yourself.

The healthy person may apply this treatment to himself, unaided, after a little practice upon himself. Try it with dry sheets first, and then take the regular treatment, after you have learned to adjust the coverings. There is no great secret to it—just a little knack, that's all.

CHAPTER X.

OTHER VALUABLE METHODS.

In addition to the use and application of water along the lines of the several methods and principles of application mentioned in the previous chapters, there are a number of other valuable Hindu methods adapted for use in special cases to which we wish to direct your attention. We shall endeavor to give you the cream of the methods in a consise form leaving out the non-essentials and an extended discussion concerning these several forms of treatment.

Fomentations. A Fomentation is a warm or hot application to a part of the body, for the purpose of relieving pain, relaxing muscles, relieving spasms, gripings, headaches, etc. They are generally given in the shape of cloths soaked in hot water—as hot as can be borne by the patient—wrung nearly dry, and then placed in a handkerchief or thin cloth and applied so that the part may be steamed.

Hot Fomentations are wonderfully efficacious when applied locally to relieve severe pains. They act, not as does the pack by drawing to the surface the waste matter to be eliminated; but, on the contrary, by drawing an extra supply of blood to the surface, thus raising the local temperature of the part and relieving a congested condition, thus dispersing the abnormal condition causing the pain, and also acting as a sedative and relaxant.

The following is the method usually employed by the best practitioners. Take a towel which has been well soaked in water as hot as can be borne by the patient, and then folded in two or three folds—if you have a soft flannel on hand, use it in place of the towel. Then take the soaked folded towel, and enclose it in another towel, which also must be folded around the first one. Then apply to the affected part, and leave it there until it begins to cool. When it cools, replace it with another similar application. Repeat this several times, until relief is obtained. This treatment is especially useful in cases of neuralgia; pains in the stomach; pains in the kidneys; headache, etc.

WATER BANDAGES OR COMPRESSES. Bandages of cloths folded and soaked in water, either hot or cold, are used quite frequently in the Water Cure. In the cases of Hot Water Bandages, there is a double effect, the water acting along the same lines as the Wet Pack, drawing out the foul matter from the system, and at the same time relieving, and relaxing, as in the case of the Hot Fomentation. In the case of Cold Water Bandages, a stimulating, invigorating effect is produced. The Cold Water Bandage is used when it is desirable to reduce inflammation.

Hot Water Bandages are supplied in a similar manner to the Hot Fomentation, except that the wet cloth is applied directly upon the skin, and is not enclosed in another towel.

Cold Water Bandages are applied as follows: Take a napkin, handkerchief, or small towel, and soak it in cold water, folding so as to adjust to the affected part. Over the Bandage carefully place several folds of soft, dry, warm flannel, in such a manner as to practically "seal up" the Bandage so that no outside air can reach the part. Allow the bandage to remain until it becomes too dry, and then replace with another similar one. In this treatment, the patient will experience a shock at the first application of the cold bandage, which feeling, however, will quickly disappear, to be followed by the natural reaction as the blood rushes to the surface, when a comfortable, soothing warm glow will be experienced.

Cold Water Bandages are applied in cases of many different forms of pain by the practitioners of the Water Cure. The relief and effect, however, is only local and the treatment should be supplemented by Flushing the Colon, etc., in order to remove the cause of the trouble. It may be applied to the throat, chest, or abdomen, according to the necessities of the case, and the seat of the pain. When applied to the chest or abdomen, a larger towel may be used, which will necessitate a correspondingly larger covering in order to "seal up" the bandage.

FOOT BATHS. These foot baths form an important part of the general treatment of the practitioner of the Water Cure, and are also quite well known to the old fashioned mother of a large family who has had many occasions in which she has demonstrated the value of the same. They are of two kinds: (1) The Hot Foot Bath; and (2) The Cold Foot Bath.

The Hot Foot Bath acts in the direction of drawing the blood from the head, and also as a sedative and quieter of the nervous system. They are found very useful in the cases of headache, pains in the head or neck, neuralgia, cramps, congestion, etc. They are applied by placing the feet in a bucket of hot water reaching up over the ankles. The knees, legs and bucket should be protected from the outside air by means of a blanket placed around the legs of the patient, well tucked around him. The feet should be kept in the water from five to fifteen minutes, according to the requirements of the case, and the state of the patient. It is well to finish the treatment by pouring cool water over them afterward, then rubbing them dry with some friction, and slapping, and then wrapping them up well in dry warm coverings.

The Cold Foot Bath is a wonderful bracer, and its practice will harden the system and render one immune from colds, etc. It freshens up the entire system after a day's work, particularly after one has been standing or walking much during the day, and it brings a sense of relief, rest and vigor which is quite grateful to the tired person. It is conducive to a good night's sleep, and is advisable in cases of insomnia. It is a cure for cold feet. Many forms of headache will also yield to this treatment, and many weak women have been strengthened by its use during the proper time of the month, in such cases it is of course well to omit the cold foot bath during time of menstruation. The Cold Foot Bath is applied by placing the feet in a bucket of cold water reaching up to the ankles or over. The feet should be kept in the water from one to three minutes, depending upon the patient's feelings and tastes in the matter. Finish the treatment by a vigorous rubbing of the feet, accompanied by manipulation and slapping.

SPECIAL APPLICATIONS. Cold Water applied to the outer "private parts" at night before retiring, or in the morning upon rising, and then followed by a vigorous, stimulating rubbing and drying, will be found very invigorating. In India there are many cases in which sexual vitality has been preserved until very old age, or restored when once apparently lost, by this simple method. The secret consists in the increased circulation to the parts, and the consequent increased tone and vigor imparted. The very intimate connection between the sexual organism, and the entire nervous system, will result in an improved general condition where sexual vitality is preserved in its normal condition. In fact, this is one of the true purposes of sexual vitality —the invigoration of the entire system, due to natural vigor and refraining from excesses and dissipation—those who desire sex vitality only to dissipate and waste it in excesses are as foolish as those who drink strong liquors in order to give them strength. A word to the wise is sufficient in this case, we hope.

The Hindus practice a "wash-off" system regularly, in addition to their regular baths. This system consists in washing the body, from the waist down to the feet, by means of a sponge bath, or similar method—every night before retiring; and a similar process applied to the body, from the waist up to the neck, every morning before dressing. This apparently simple method has been followed with excellent results by many Europeans and Americans who have learned it, and they report that it gives them a good quiet restful night's sleep, and a vigorous, active vitality in the morning when they start out for the day's work. Try it for yourself.

IN CONCLUSION.

In this little book we have given you a number of simple, practical methods of applying the "Hindu-Yogi Water Cure," which have been in use in India and surrounding countries for many centuries. So simple are these methods, and so common is their use in those countries, that the simple folk of those lands would be greatly surprised to learn that it was necessary to instruct anyone in their use. They regard these methods as almost instinctive, and as natural to the race as walking, breathing, or sleeping. To think that people should be required to be taught the natural use of water would seem as preposterous to them as that people should need to be taught how to breathe—and yet instruction in both of these things have been found necessary by the Western peoples, whose "civilization" has led them so far away from Nature that they have forgotten the first instinctive teachings of the Great Mother of All.

We trust that you will not allow the extreme simplicity of these methods to prejudice you against them, or to prevent your use of them. Do not make this mistake. Trust the instinctive knowledge of these people of the Far East who live very close indeed to Nature, and who trust to her loving teachings. It is true that in the great cities of India the people have departed from their ancient customs and habits, but in the country away from the cities the Hindus live as they lived centuries ago, close to Nature and receiving her benefits. One has to pay the price for the advantages of "civilization"—and that price is often Disease and Weakness. But if the original Natural Methods of Physical Well-Being are adhered to, one may have both "the penny of Health and the Cake of Civilization." We trust that this little book will lead many to the right and natural path of living. Water, Air and Sunshine—these are Nature's three best gifts to Man. Let him appreciate them, and use them as he should. These three Natural

Remedies would almost abolish Disease, were they properly used by the race. But at least, YOU may use them, whether or not others do.

FINIS.